READ 15 MINUTES AND YOU CAN SAVE A LIFE

BLS AND CPR IN THE STREET

Dr. Omar Shakoree

Dr. Omar M. G. Shakoree
SHO A&E Surgery
Department of Emergency
Sulaymaniah teaching hospital
Sulaymaniah, Iraq.
E-mail: omarshakoree@gmail.com
www.facebook.com/Dr.OmarShakoree

For my family

For my paients

For the people in need

For a life saving

Omar Shakoree

AIMS OF THIS BOOK

- To know what we mean of BLS

- Why BLS is important

- Who can do BLS

- For which person you do BLS

- When to activate BLS

- Steps

- Summary

- Chain of survival

- Common Scenario you may face

- When to stop

- What's new in AHA

WHAT WE MEAN OF BLS

- BLS is the foundation for saving lives after cardiac arrest

- It is a type of care that first-responder, healthcare provider and public safety professionals can provide it.

- first-responder can be any person who's age +12 years and know what is the BLS and its step

- BLS consist of a series of sequential assessments and actions, which are illustrated and simplified in this course.

WHY BLS IS IMPORTANT

- Sudden cardiac arrest remains a leading cause of death in the United States and allover the world.

- Seventy percent of out-of-hospital cardiac arrests occur in the home, streets and a places outside the hospitals.

- survival can approach 50% if you know how to do BLS.

I AM TEACHING YOU THE BLS, WHY ?

- I will do my best efforts to make this type of actions easy and applicable for you to do it, regardless your age and where you are, but why ?

- Believe me

- You may safe your family

- You may safe your friend

- You may safe a stranger

- You may safe my life one day

- It is about life saving

WHO ? FOR WHOM ? WHEN ?

Who can do BLS ?

Any person aged over 12 years can do it if trained, not only the medical or social staff.

For any person you do BLS?

You will do it for any victim aged over 8 years who get a sudden collapse in the street or home.

When to activate BLS ?

BLS must be activated whenever you witnesses a victim aged over 8 years who get a sudden collapse (fainting attack, LOC) in the street or home and unresponsive.

STEPS OF BLS

- There are a seven steps for performing BLS

- Steps of BLS consist of a series of sequential assessments and actions, which are illustrated and simplified in BLS algorithm

- Steps are easy for all types of rescuers to learn, remember, and perform.

STEP ONE

Ensure scene safety

- How ?

- Look around the victim

- Any gas, electrical line and fire ?

- Tell the people to give you a space and take the victim to safe area

- Go to step 2

STEP TWO

Assess responsiveness

How ?

Shaking the victim

Tapping on the chest

If unresponsive

continue to step 3.

Assessing responsiveness

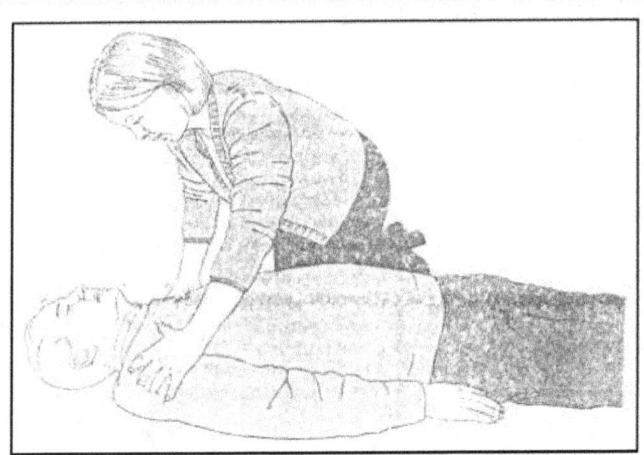

TAP ON THE SHOULDER & SHOUT "are you all right"

STEP THREE

Call 911 and get activate the BLS care

If possible, call for an assistant to do so.

If no assistant is available and underlying etiology is asphyxia (i.e., drowning), call 911.

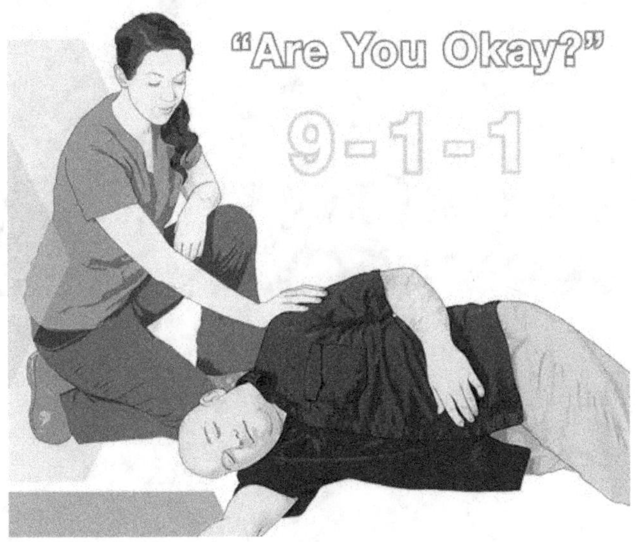

STEP FOUR

Position victim and Open the airway

Head tilt/chin left (B) and jaw thrust(C).
Maintain cervical spine immobilization if trauma.

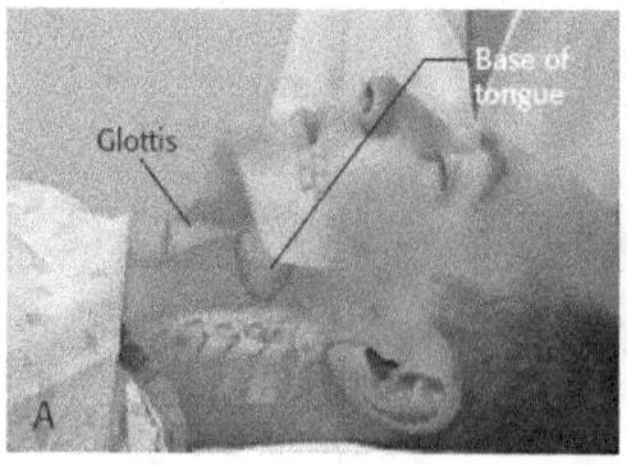

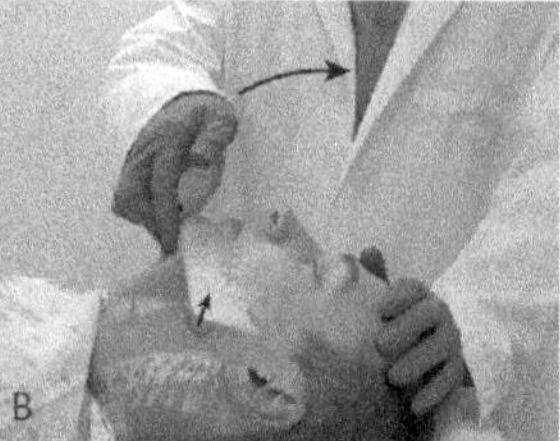

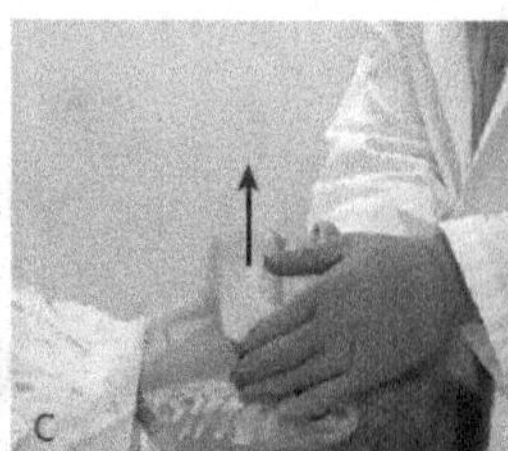

STEP FIVE

Pulse Check and look for breathing

check for a pulse, limiting the time to no more than 10 seconds to avoid   delay in initiation of chest compressions.

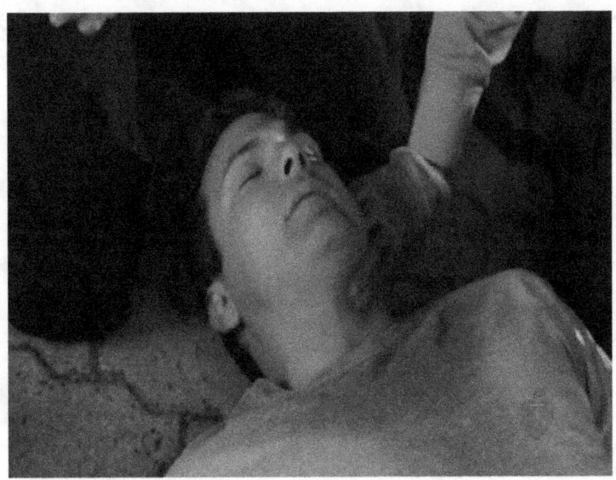

STEP SIX

Begin CPR by closed chest compressions and ventilations.

- Push hard, fast, and deep
- 100 compressions/min
- Compress 4–5 cm (~2 in.).
- Allow for complete chest recoil and minimize interruptions.
- Ratio of 30 compressions to 2 breaths (30:2)
- For 5 cycles
- Breaths should be of sufficient volume to cause visible chest rise.

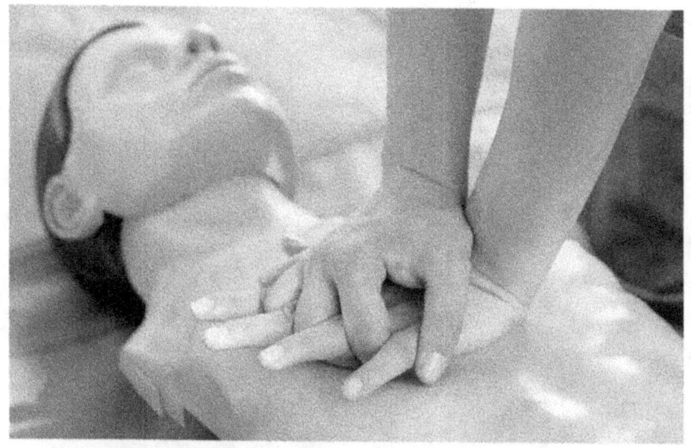

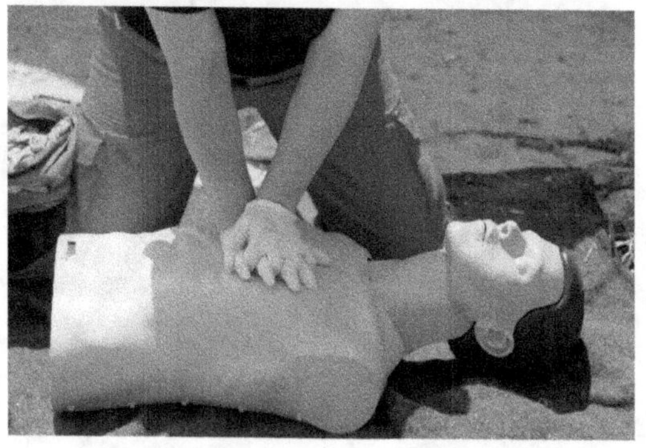

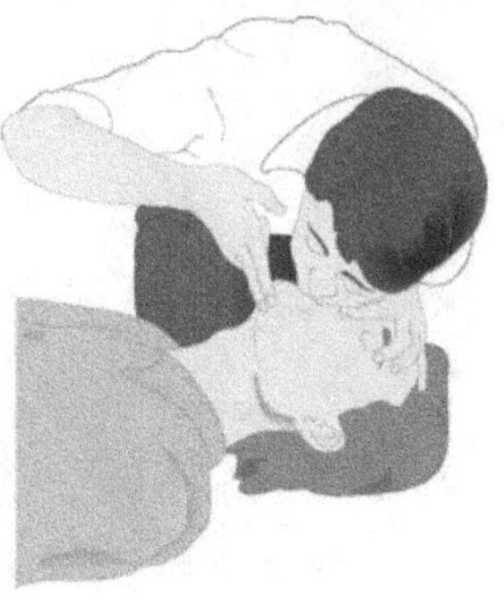

STEP SEVEN

Use the AED defibrillator when available and indicated.

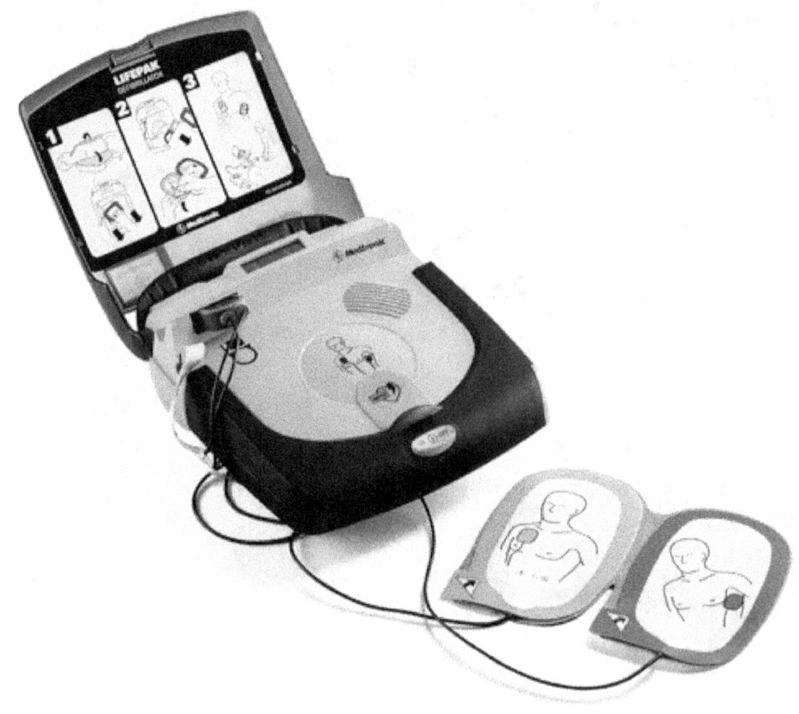

SUMMERY AHA FIGURE

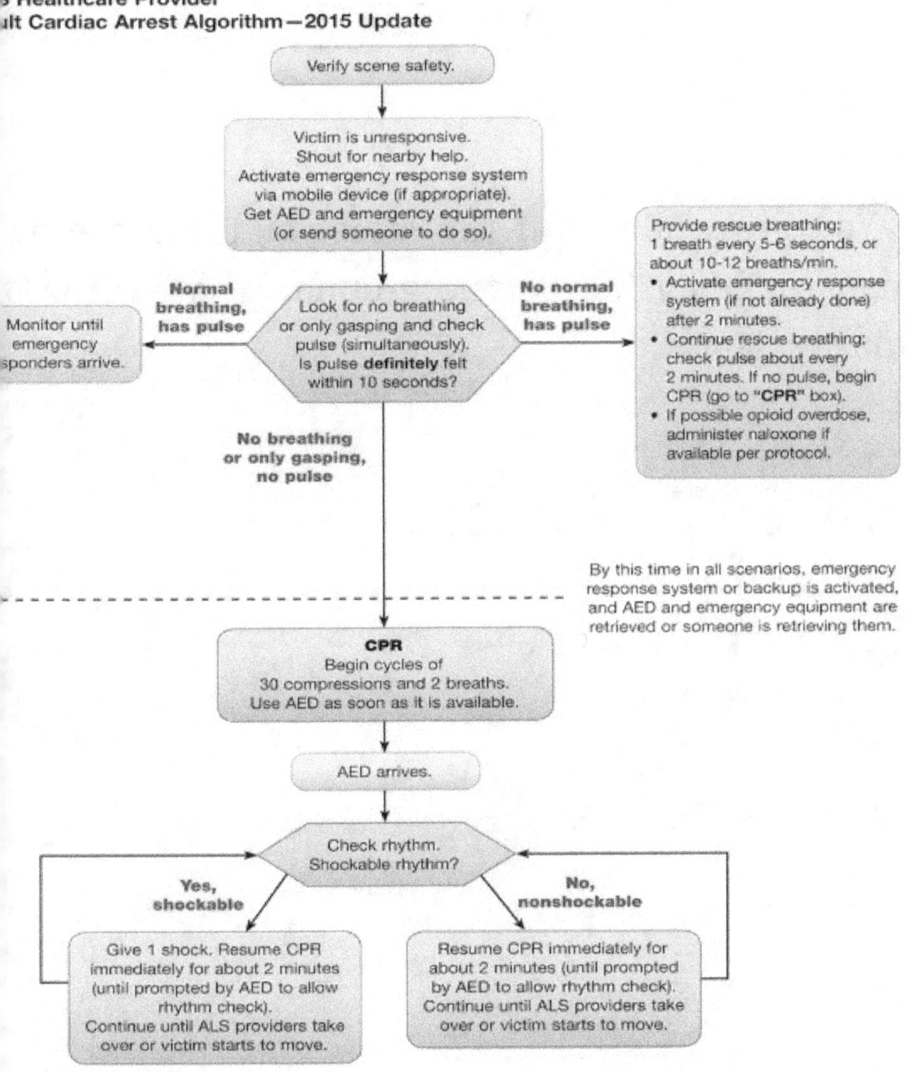

COMMON SCENARIO YOU MAY FACE

You are walking in the street and you see a man suddenly fall on the ground, what will be your response ?

1) Ensure scene safety
2) Check responsiveness
3) Call 911
4) Position and Open airway
5) Check pulse
6) Start CPR 30:2
7) Use AED if available

WHEN TO STOP ?

- Don't stop unless the EMS team arrived and take care of the victim.

- You are the life rescuer for this victim

CHAIN OF SURVIVAL

Early access to the victim

Early CPR

Early defibrillation

Early advanced care

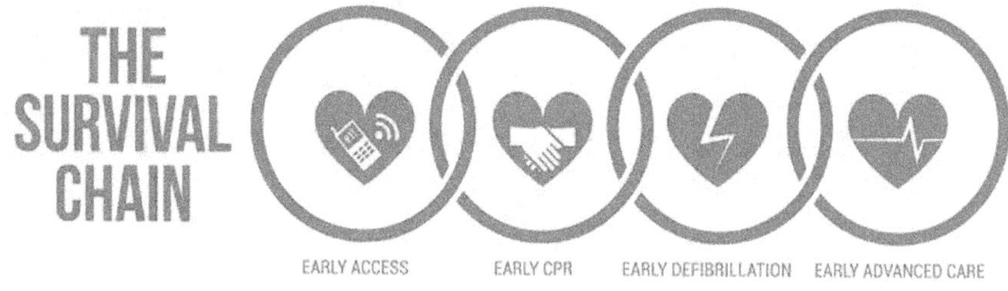

WHAT'S NEW IN AHA??

Hands – Only CPR

- Every minute CPR is delayed, a victim's chance of survival decreases by 10%.
- Immediate CPR from someone nearby can double – even triple – their chance of survival.
- Remember these two steps if you see a teen or adult suddenly collapse

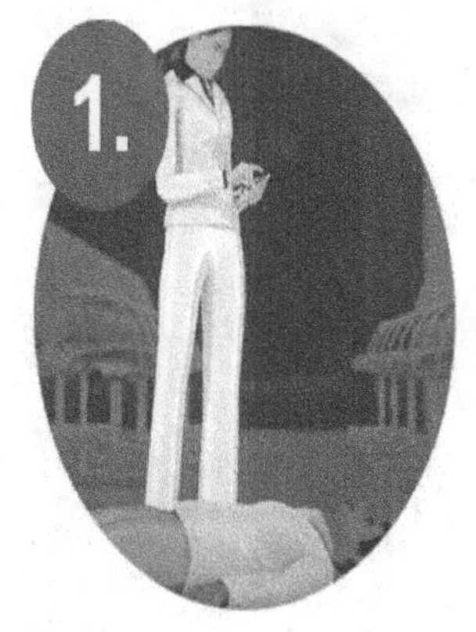

Call

your local emergency response number

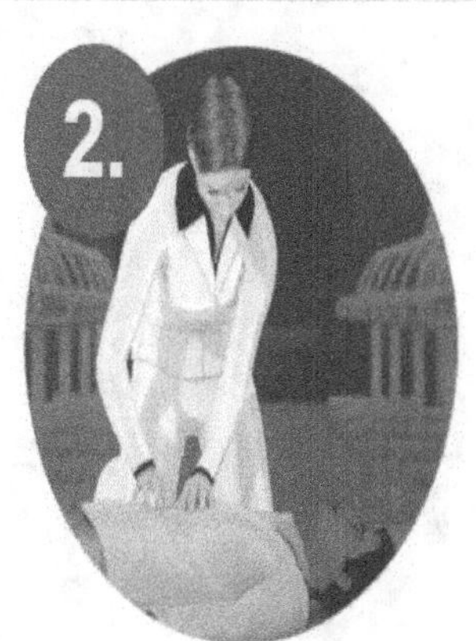

Push

hard and fast in the center of the chest

LAST THING

Online course study and videos are available in many websites you can check for that just type BLS basic life support and learn more.

My online course will be available as soon as possible and you can roll in.

You can contact me and I will guide you.

CONTACT INFORMATION

E-mail: omarshakoree@gmail.com
www.youtube.com/omarshakoree
www.facebook.com/Dr.OmarShakoree

Dr. Omar Shakoree

www.ingramcontent.com/pod-product-compliance
Lightning Source LLC
Chambersburg PA
CBHW050800250726
48662CB00005B/2332